- **Book Name**

- Energy Medicine

- **Title**

- Energize Your Life: The Ultimate Guide to Energy Medicine

- **Written by**

- Sam Berman

Table of Contents

Chapter 1: "The Essence of Energy Medicine"

- We will investigate the basic ideas that guide the use of energy medicine in this introductory chapter. We explore the fundamental ideas and historical foundations that have influenced the development of this revolutionary methodology.

- Origins and Historical Views: We start by tracing the history of energy medicine by looking at age-old healing customs from many cultures. We reveal the common thread of identifying and assisting with the essential life energy that animates all living things, found in both Ayurveda and Traditional Chinese Medicine.

-

1.2 The Life Force All Around Us: The Foundation of Energy The idea of a universal life force, or energy, that permeates all living things is the foundation of medicine. We look at the various ways that other cultures have understood this energy—qi in Chinese medicine, prana in Ayurveda, for example—and how it forms the basis for knowledge of health and well-being.

- The Subtle Energy Body: The notion of the subtle energy body is introduced, building upon the notion of the universal life force. Investigating the chakra system and meridians is part of this, as they are essential to comprehending the movement of energy throughout the human body. Readers will learn more about the connections between the spiritual, emotional, and physical facets of health through this investigation.

- The Transition to Contemporary Views: Next, we look at how energy medicine has developed in the current day, emphasizing the fusion of traditional knowledge with cutting-edge scientific research. This part promotes a thorough grasp of the area by bridging the gap between conventional wisdom and recent research.

- The Holistic Nature of Energy Medicine: Stressing the holistic aspect of energy medicine, this chapter comes to a close. This approach takes into account how physical, emotional, and spiritual well-being are intertwined rather than seeing the body as a collection of separate parts. Now that they have a basic understanding of energy medicine, readers can move on to more in-depth discussions of real-world uses and life-changing events in later chapters.

- # Chapter 2: "The Body's Energy Blueprint"

- This is a critical chapter where we decipher the workings of the body's energy system and offer a clear picture of the blueprint that controls the movement of life force within. Readers learn how these energy channels affect mental, emotional, and physical health as we examine the meridians and chakras.

- 2.1 Charting the Meridians: In this section, we explore the idea of meridians, which are energy lines that carry vital life force. We examine how these pathways function as channels for energy distribution and balance, connecting different organs and systems, with inspiration from traditional Chinese medicine.

-

2.2 Chakras: Energy Wheels: The investigation also includes the chakra system, a network of energy centers vital to preserving the body's balance. The seven primary chakras—each linked to certain facets of physical, emotional, and spiritual well-being—become clearer to readers.

- 2.3 Energy Disproportions and Obstructions: We look at how energy flow imbalances and obstructions might affect general health, building on the concepts of meridians and chakras. In order to enable readers to identify and resolve possible problems within their own energy blueprint, this section examines the telltale indications and symptoms of interrupted energy.
- 2.4 Harmony Restoration: Methods and Approaches:
This section focuses on doable methods for bringing the body's energy system back into harmony and balance. The introduction of methods like acupressure, acupuncture, and other energy-based therapies gives readers the skills they need to correct energy imbalances and advance wellbeing.
- 2.5 Blending Western and Eastern Viewpoints: We integrate Eastern and Western ideas into the body's energy blueprint to provide a

comprehensive understanding. Readers are given a more sophisticated understanding of the intricate relationship between the physical and energetic aspects of health by making linkages between traditional practices and contemporary scientific knowledge.

- 2.6 Personal Energy Evaluation: This section walks readers through a personal energy evaluation to help them become more self-aware. Through comprehension of their individual energy blueprint, readers can customize their energy medicine practices to target particular requirements, promoting a customized and efficient approach to overall well-being.

- 2.7 Beginning Practical Application: The chapter ends with an invitation for readers to put their newly acquired information to use. Setting the groundwork for practical investigation, the exercises and suggestions encourage readers to actively interact with their body's energy design and begin on a path to improved vitality and balance.

Chapter 3: "Breath work and Energy Alignment"

- We explore the fundamental relationship between breath and energy in this enlightening chapter, and we use conscious breathwork to unleash the possibility for healing and balance. The examination of several breathwork methods is facilitated for the readers, revealing the ways in which deliberate breathing can affect and harmonize the body's energy.

-

  3.1 The Breath as a Conduit of Energy: The breath is introduced as a potent energy conduit at the beginning of the chapter. We go into the age-old knowledge that acknowledges the breath as a conduit between the energetic and physical domains, emphasizing its function in promoting the life force's distribution throughout the body.

- 3.2 Pranayama and Traditional Breathing Techniques:

  Inspired by age-old techniques like yoga's

Pranayama, readers are exposed to particular breathwork techniques that have been practiced for ages. We examine the ways in which these practices support mental clarity, energy alignment, and general wellbeing.

- 3.3 Mindful Breathing to Lower Stress: This section examines the transforming power of conscious breathing in stress reduction. Readers discover how deliberate breathing exercises can trigger the body's relaxation response, reducing the negative effects of stress on the physical and mental levels.

- 3.4 Aligning with the Cycles of Nature: This chapter delves deeper into the topic of coordinating breathwork with the body's and the environment's natural cycles. Gaining an awareness of how breath links us to life's cyclical patterns cultivates a stronger feeling of balance and resonance with the energetic flow both inside and outside of ourselves.

- 3.5 Energetic Breath Practices: This section introduces readers to breath techniques meant to affect the body's energy system. Readers can explore and incorporate the wide toolkit provided in this part, which ranges from stimulating tactics to cleansing breaths, into their daily lives.

- 3.6 Mindful Breath in Meditation: This section examines the relationship between breath and meditation, highlighting the way that mindful breathing can lead to increased consciousness and a deeper spiritual connection. Readers are guided through practical exercises that help them integrate breath work into their meditation practices for a more comprehensive and meaningful experience.

- 3.7 Customized Breathwork Schedules: This section offers advice on establishing customized routines so that readers can customize breathwork to meet their own requirements. Since every person has a different energetic landscape, readers are advised to try out various breathwork techniques to see which ones work best for them.

- 3.8 Integration into Daily Life: To wrap up the chapter, several real-world examples of how to incorporate conscious breathwork into everyday life are provided. In order to maintain a sense of vitality and balance, readers learn how to use their breath to continuously align their energy, whether they are working, exercising, or relaxing.

- # Chapter 4: "The Power of Visualization and Intention"

- This chapter explores the transforming field of intention-setting and imagery as a means of releasing the creative potential of the mind. The investigation of how focused intention and mental imagery can affect the body's energy, opening doors for healing, manifestation, and personal development, is led for readers.

- 4.1 The Mind-Body Connection: This chapter opens with a discussion of the close relationship that exists between the mind and the body. The science underlying the mind-body connection is explored by readers, who learn how mental images and thoughts can affect the energy field and physiological reactions.

-

4.2 Visualization Methods: A range of visualization methods aimed at improving the body's energy flow are presented to the readers. This area offers useful activities that enable people to actively use their imagination for healing and balance, ranging from creative visualization to guided imagery.

- 4.3 The Intentional Role: Intention-setting is discussed, and its importance in focusing energy on desired results is emphasized. By understanding the power of intention to shape one's energetic experiences and general well-being, readers gain the ability to create intentions that are both clear and constructive.

- 4.4 Visualization for Healing: The use of visualization for healing is the main topic of this section. The impact of vivid health, harmony, and balance visualization on the body's energy and its ability to support mental, physical, and emotional well-being is examined by readers.

- 4.5 Energy Alignment and Manifestation: Expanding upon the potency of intention, readers learn how vision functions as a manifestation technique. People develop a sense of purpose and empowerment by learning to mold their energetic reality by lining up their mental images with desired results.

- 4.6 Chakra Balancing with Visualization: This chapter delves into particular uses, such as balancing chakras using visualization. In order to promote total energetic alignment and vitality, readers are led through exercises to picture the vivid and harmonious functioning of each chakra.

- 4.7 Guided Meditation for Intention: In this part, readers examine how meditation, intention, and imagery work together. In order to assist people in developing their practice and improving their capacity to concentrate and direct their intention toward life-changing events, guided meditation activities have been devised.

- 4.8 Integrating Visualization into Daily Life: Readers can easily incorporate intention-setting and visualization into their daily routines by following the helpful advice and recommendations offered. Readers are invited to incorporate these activities, which are widely accessible, into their lives in order to make them more enjoyable and enriching.

- 4.9 Fostering a Positive Mindset: The importance of a positive mindset in energy alignment is emphasized in this chapter's conclusion. Readers who adopt a positive and upbeat mindset acknowledge the transforming potential found in the power of intention and imagery, and they also set the stage for continued energetic well-being.

Chapter 5: "Hands-On Healing: The Art of Energy Touch"

- We dig into the complex art of hands-on healing in this enlightening chapter, where we examine the profound technique of utilizing touch to affect and balance the body's energy. With a focus on both traditional and modern techniques, this chapter provides readers with an overview of the fundamentals and practices of hands-on healing, enabling them to connect with and work with healing energies in both themselves and others.

- 5.1 The Energetic Exchange via Touch: The first step in the process is realizing how important touch is to energy healing. It presents the idea that touch is a vehicle for the exchange of energy as well as a physical experience. The connection that is made possible by hands-on healing enables readers to manipulate and transfer healing energy.

-

5.2 Reiki: The Energy of the Universal Life Force

A thorough examination of Reiki is presented, providing insight into this Japanese healing technique that uses the hands to transfer life force energy from all around the world. The chapter gives readers a basic grasp of this widely used hands-on healing technique by going over Reiki concepts, hand placements, and the attunement procedure.

- 5.3 Therapeutic Touch and Healing Hands: In this section, therapeutic touch—a mindful, hands-on healing technique—is introduced. Through the exploration of energy sensing and manipulation techniques, readers are equipped to provide therapeutic touch for their own well-being as well as to support the healing process of others.

- 5.4 Chakra Balancing with Direct Healing Touch: The chapter explores particular uses, emphasizing therapeutic touch for chakra balancing. Methods for using touch to evaluate and harmonize the body's energy centers are discussed, promoting a balanced flow of energy and correcting imbalances that could show up as mental or physical problems.

- 5.5 Energy Transfer and Intention: This section focuses on the significance of intention in practical healing. The chapter focuses on how the focused intention of the healer affects the energy that is transferred during touch. The useful activities in this book help readers develop a conscious and purposeful approach to hands-on healing, which will improve the efficacy of their work.

- 5.6 Using Hands-On Healing to Reduce Stress: It is demonstrated how gentle touch can trigger the body's relaxation response, highlighting the transforming power of hands-on healing in stress reduction. Readers learn how practical methods support equilibrium and serenity on an energetic and bodily level.

- 5.7 Methods for Self-Healing: This section presents practical healing practices for self-care, empowering readers to take an active role in their own well-being. Through hands-on exercises, people learn how to release tension, encourage relaxation, and maintain their general energetic well-being.

- 5.8 Hands-on Healing Integrated Into Holistic Wellness: Useful advice is given on how hands-on healing fits in with a holistic wellness regimen. It is recommended that readers consider this practice as an auxiliary tool that can improve overall health when paired with other energy medicine methods, mindfulness exercises, and lifestyle decisions.
- 5.9 The Art and Ethics of Energy Touch: This section looks at the subtleties and ethical issues surrounding hands-on healing as it wraps up the chapter. As a result, readers are better able to see the value of decency, permission, and honesty in the practice, which promotes a responsible and balanced approach to the practice of energy contact. This chapter provides a thorough introduction to the transformative art of hands-on healing, including theoretical understanding as well as real-world applications for individuals interested in pursuing this path.

Chapter 6: "Crystals and Energy Resonance"

- We dig into the complex art of hands-on healing in this enlightening chapter, where we examine the profound technique of utilizing touch to affect and balance the body's energy. With a focus on both traditional and modern techniques, this chapter provides readers with an overview of the fundamentals and practices of hands-on healing, enabling them to connect with and work with healing energies in both themselves and others.

- 5.1 The Energetic Exchange via Touch: The first step in the process is realizing how important touch is to energy healing. It presents the idea that touch is a vehicle for the exchange of energy as well as a physical experience. The connection that is made possible by hands-on healing enables readers to manipulate and transfer healing energy.

-

5.2 Reiki: The Energy of the Universal Life Force

A thorough examination of Reiki is presented, providing insight into this Japanese healing technique that uses the hands to transfer life force energy from all around the world. The chapter gives readers a basic grasp of this widely used hands-on healing technique by going over Reiki concepts, hand placements, and the attunement procedure.

- 5.3 Therapeutic Touch and Healing Hands: In this section, therapeutic touch—a mindful, hands-on healing technique—is introduced. Through the exploration of energy sensing and manipulation techniques, readers are equipped to provide therapeutic touch for their own well-being as well as to support the healing process of others.

- 5.4 Chakra Balancing with Direct Healing Touch: The chapter explores particular uses, emphasizing therapeutic touch for chakra balancing. Methods for using touch to evaluate and harmonize the body's energy centers are discussed, promoting a balanced flow of energy and correcting imbalances that could show up as mental or physical problems.

- 5.5 Energy Transfer and Intention: This section focuses on the significance of intention in practical healing. The chapter focuses on how the focused intention of the healer affects the energy that is transferred during touch. The useful activities in this book help readers develop a conscious and purposeful approach to hands-on healing, which will improve the efficacy of their work.

- 5.6 Using Hands-On Healing to Reduce Stress: It is demonstrated how gentle touch can trigger the body's relaxation response, highlighting the transforming power of hands-on healing in stress reduction. Readers learn how practical methods support equilibrium and serenity on an energetic and bodily level.

- 5.7 Methods for Self-Healing: This section presents practical healing practices for self-care, empowering readers to take an active role in their own well-being. Through hands-on exercises, people learn how to release tension, encourage relaxation, and maintain their general energetic well-being.

- 5.8 Hands-on Healing Integrated Into Holistic Wellness: Useful advice is given on how hands-on healing fits in with a holistic wellness regimen. It is recommended that readers consider this practice as an auxiliary tool that can improve overall health when paired with other energy medicine methods, mindfulness exercises, and lifestyle decisions.

- 5.9 The Art and Ethics of Energy Touch: This section looks at the subtleties and ethical issues surrounding hands-on healing as it wraps up the chapter. As a result, readers are better able to see the value of decency, permission, and honesty in the practice, which promotes a responsible and balanced approach to the practice of energy contact. This chapter provides a thorough introduction to the transformative art of hands-on healing, including theoretical understanding as well as real-world applications for individuals interested in pursuing this path.

Chapter 7: "Sound Therapy and Vibrational Healing"

- 7.1 The Power of Sound in Healing: The first point made in this chapter is the natural ability of sound to be a healing medium. As they examine the historical and cultural applications of sound in healing, readers come to understand the widespread belief that music has the power to affect people's experiences on a physical, emotional, and spiritual level.

-

  7.2 The Body and Vibrational Resonance: In-depth, we investigate the idea of vibrational resonance and the relationship between sound waves and the body's energetic field. The science of vibrational healing is explained to readers, who learn how sound waves can infiltrate and affect tissues, cells, and energy centers.

- 7.3 Instruments of Healing: A range of instruments, from tuning forks and crystal bowls to singing bowls and gongs, are offered as part of sound therapy. The distinctive features of each instrument are explained to the reader, along with how they might be used to produce particular vibrational frequencies for medicinal effects.

- 7.4 Chakra Tuning and Sound Alignment: Sound therapy's useful applications for chakra tuning are examined. In order to promote a harmonious flow of energy and correct imbalances within the energetic system, readers learn how to use particular sound frequencies to balance and align the body's energy centers.

- 7.5 Sound Bath Experiences: This chapter delves into the world of immersive sound baths, which engulf people in a symphony of healing noises. The transforming power of sound baths for unwinding, lowering stress levels, and achieving energy alignment is revealed to readers.

- 7.6 Voice as a Healing Instrument: Research is done on the use of the human voice as a potent healing tool. Readers learn about vocal, chanting, and tone practices that can be used for others' energetic well-being as well as self-healing.

- 7.7 Solfeggio Scale and Healing Frequencies: This section delves into the investigation of healing frequencies, which encompasses the Solfeggio scale. To understand how particular musical tones can aid in vibrational healing, readers dig into the history of solfeggio frequencies and their alleged therapeutic benefits.

- 7.8 Sound Meditation and Mindful Listening: Using sound meditation techniques, readers are guided by practical activities to develop mindfulness and strengthen their connection to the restorative vibrations of sound. This section invites readers to investigate the meditative properties of music and how it might improve mental and emotional health.

- 7.9 Including Sound Therapy in Everyday Life: Useful advice is given on how to include sound therapy in everyday life. Readers learn how to create a space that fosters continuous vibrational healing, from setting up a personal sound sanctuary to incorporating sound rituals into everyday activities.

- 7.10 Investigating the Soundscapes of Healing: This chapter's encouragement to delve deeper into the wide and varied realm of soundscapes for healing comes to a close. Readers are encouraged to embrace the dynamic and approachable nature of sound therapy within the larger framework of energy medicine, whether through participating in sound healing sessions, developing their own sound rituals, or combining sound into already-existing wellness practices. This chapter provides a thorough overview of sound therapy and its ability to improve the energetic components of well-being, making it a useful resource for both novices and enthusiasts.

- # Chapter 8: "Quantum Healing and Energy Medicine"

- We take a deep dive into the concepts and practices that underlie the concept of quantum healing in this insightful chapter, which explores the nexus between energy medicine and quantum physics. By learning more about the quantum aspect of reality and how it connects to the body's energy, readers will be able to better comprehend the mind-body connection in the context of energy medicine.

- 8.1 The Quantum Nature of Reality: This chapter starts out by exploring the basic ideas of quantum physics, introducing readers to the idea of a quantum field and the idea that all matter is related. We investigate how conventional ideas of reality are challenged by the concepts of superposition and entanglement, providing the foundation for comprehending the quantum nature of healing.

- 8.2 Quantum Entanglement and Histories of Healing: This section presents readers with the idea of quantum entanglement and how it relates to energy medicine. A better understanding of the potential healing links within the quantum field is fostered by exploring the interconnection of particles—even at a distance—as a metaphor for the interconnectedness of the human experience.

- 8.3 Quantum Awareness and the Mind-Body Link: The investigation also includes consciousness's function in the quantum world. Readers learn how the energetic dynamics of the body are influenced by consciousness, intention, and observation. The potential for deliberate attention to influence healing at the quantum level is revealed when the mind-body link is analyzed through the prism of quantum consciousness.

- 8.4 Quantum Healing Modalities: This section introduces the useful uses of quantum theory in energy therapy. The concepts of resonance and intention are used by quantum healing therapies like quantum touch and matrix energetics to promote healing on an energy level.

- 8.5 The Function of Vibration and Frequency: This chapter examines the function of vibration and frequency in the quantum healing paradigm. The ability of particular frequencies and vibrations to affect the quantum field and aid in reestablishing harmony and balance in the body's energy is explained to readers.

- 8.6 Energy Medicine and the Observer Effect: This section discusses the application of the Observer Effect, a fundamental idea in quantum physics, to the field of energy medicine. By emphasizing the importance of consciousness and intention in the healing process, readers learn how the act of observation, whether carried out by a practitioner or by the individual themselves, can affect the results of energetic treatments.

- 8.7 Quantum Biofeedback and Energetic Assessment: The investigation of quantum biofeedback technologies and their function in energetic assessment is covered in this chapter. In order to bridge the gap between quantum ideas and real-world applications for evaluation and intervention, readers are introduced to instruments that make use of quantum principles in order to offer insights into the body's energy field.

- 8.8 Integrating Quantum Healing into Energy Practices: This section offers helpful advice on how to incorporate the concepts of quantum healing into currently used energy medicine procedures. It is suggested that readers accept the quantum viewpoint as an additional framework that deepens their comprehension of the energetic basis of health and wellbeing.

- 8.9 Investigating Quantum Opportunities for Personal Development: To wrap up the chapter, readers are urged to investigate quantum opportunities for personal development. In their quest for improved energy well-being, people are encouraged to embrace the transforming potential of quantum principles, whether via mindfulness, intention-setting, or investigating quantum healing treatments. In the framework of energy medicine, this chapter acts as a link between the quantum world and the real-world implementation of quantum healing.

Chapter 9: "Holistic Approaches to Energy Medicine"

- We examine the holistic aspects of energy medicine in this integrative chapter, highlighting the connections between different modalities and lifestyle factors that affect overall health. Readers will learn how energy medicine can be effortlessly combined with movement, mindfulness, and nutrition to promote a comprehensive and synergistic approach to holistic health.

- 9.1 The Holistic Paradigm: In the framework of energy medicine, the chapter defines the holistic paradigm from the outset. The notion that the body, mind, and spirit are interrelated and that treating the whole person rather than just specific symptoms leads to optimal health and vitality is explored by readers.

-

  9.2 Nutrition and Energetic Nourishment: An examination of nutrition's function in energy medicine is conducted. Readers explore the idea of energetically rich foods and their potential to assist the body's energy system, gaining insights into how our diets might affect our energetic balance.

- 9.3 Movement as Energy Medicine: This section introduces physical movement as a potent kind of energy medicine. The chapter looks at how energy-related activities like qigong, yoga, and tai chi can improve the body's energy flow and foster flexibility, strength, and general energetic balance.

- 9.4 Mindfulness and Energetic Presence: Emphasis is placed on the transforming power of mindfulness exercises. Readers discover how stress reduction, improved mental and emotional balance, and a stronger connection to the present moment are all achieved through techniques like mindfulness and meditation, which all contribute to energy well-being.

- 9.5 Integrative Medicine and Energy Healing: In this section, readers examine the relationship between integrative medicine and energy healing. The chapter encourages people to collaborate with healthcare providers to develop a customized, all-encompassing wellness plan, emphasizing the synergy between traditional and complementary therapies.

- 9.6 Self-Care and Energetic Hygiene Practices: There are helpful tips on how to keep your energy clean and fit self-care routines into your everyday routine. Learn how techniques like aura protection, grounding, and energy cleaning support general energetic well-being and build resilience in the face of adversity.

- 9.7 Nature as a Source of Healing Energy: This chapter explores nature's capacity for healing. Learn how spending time in the outdoors, sometimes referred to as "forest bathing" or "earthing," can have a beneficial effect on the body's energy field and encourage rest, renewal, and a feeling of connectedness to the planet.

- 9.8 Energy Medicine Retreats and Holistic Experiences: The possibility of these retreats and experiences being transformed is examined. It is recommended that readers investigate immersive and transforming settings that include a blend of mindfulness exercises, holistic activities, and energy healing treatments in order to enhance their overall wellbeing.

- 9.9 Finding a Work-Life Balance to Promote Energy Health: Useful advice on finding a work-life balance to promote energy health is given. The chapter invites readers to reflect on how their daily routines, places of employment, and recreational pursuits might either enhance or diminish their overall energy balance.

- 9.10 Fostering a Holistic Perspective for Enduring Well-Being:

The last words of the chapter exhort readers to develop a holistic mentality for long-term wellbeing. By accepting that all areas of their lives are interconnected and integrating holistic practices into their daily routines, people are motivated to set out on a path toward long-term energy balance and vitality. This chapter provides guidance for individuals who want to use energy medicine in a holistic manner, understanding the complex relationship between physical, mental, and spiritual health and the possibility of profound change when treating all three at once.

- # Chapter 10: "Embarking on Your Lifelong Energy Medicine Journey"

- This final chapter provides readers with guidance on how to use energy medicine to start a lifetime path of self-discovery and energetic well-being. This chapter provides a road map for incorporating the concepts, methods, and information covered in the book into a transforming and unique journey towards perpetual vitality.

- 10.1 Accepting Personal Empowerment: The relevance of personal empowerment in the development of energy medicine is emphasized at the outset of this chapter. It is suggested that readers acknowledge their intrinsic capacity to take an active role in their own health and well-being by consciously forming their energy environment through behaviors and decisions.

- 10.2 Building Your Customized Energy Medicine Toolkit: Useful advice is given on building a customized energy medicine toolkit. In order to build a customized toolkit for their continuing journey, readers consider the modalities, approaches, and practices presented in the book and choose the ones that best connect with them.
- 10.3 Creating Objectives and Intentions: In order to help readers develop specific intents and goals for their journey with energy medicine, the transforming power of intention is examined. Readers gain the ability to express and visualize their goals for well-being, regardless of whether they are centered on spiritual development, emotional equilibrium, or physical health.
- 10.4 Establishing Routines and Habits Every Day: There are helpful hints on how to use rituals and practices to incorporate energy medicine into daily life. The ways that readers might create routines that support their objectives and integrate energy medicine into their daily lives are explored.

- 10.5 Taking Care of the Mind, Body, and Spirit Triad:

  It emphasizes the mind-body-spirit connection's holistic character. It is recommended that readers take care of this interdependent triangle, understanding that each component's well-being affects the others. Engaging in hands-on activities helps people cultivate a harmonious relationship between their mental, physical, and spiritual aspects.

- 10.6 Lifelong Learning and Investigation: In the subject of energy medicine, readers are encouraged to adopt a mindset of lifelong learning and investigation. The chapter recognizes that the process of self-discovery is ongoing and dynamic and encourages readers to be receptive to new approaches, theories, and experiences.

- 10.7 Seeking Community and Support: Emphasis is placed on the value of community and support throughout the path of energy medicine. It is suggested that readers establish connections with people who share their interests through local clubs, online communities, or workshops.

This will promote a shared sense of inspiration, encouragement, and learning.

- 10.8 Accepting Difficulties and Rejoicing in Progress: This chapter discusses the inevitable difficulties that arise in the practice of energy medicine. Readers gain the ability to view obstacles as chances for personal development and exploration. It's stressed that acknowledging and appreciating tiny victories is crucial for staying motivated and developing an optimistic outlook.

- 10.9 Incorporating Life Transitions with Energy Medicine:
  There are helpful tips on how to incorporate energy medicine techniques into different life stages. Through professional transitions, relationship changes, or significant life events, readers learn how energy medicine may provide a stable and encouraging environment throughout these times.

- 10.10 Cultivating Gratitude and Joy: The Path Through Energy Medicine examines the transformational power of gratitude and joy as fundamental components. It is suggested that readers develop an attitude of gratitude for the current moment, which will promote optimism and fortitude in the face of life's ups and downs.

- 10.11 Sharing Your Journey and Inspiring Others: The last section of the chapter asks readers to tell others about their experiences using energy medicine. Through one-on-one interactions, writing, or community service, people are encouraged to elevate and inspire others as they travel their own journeys toward wellbeing.

- This chapter offers readers encouragement, insights, and useful tools to promote a lifetime of self-discovery, vitality, and holistic well-being as they embark on the ongoing journey of energy medicine.

www.ingramcontent.com/pod-product-compliance
Lightning Source LLC
Chambersburg PA
CBHW070226260726
48658CB00006BA/2188